AFTER YOUR JAW SURGERY

PRACTICAL AND HELPFUL INFORMATION YOU SHOULD KNOW

Jayne Flaagan

Table of Contents

CHAPTER 1

Who Can Benefit From Reading This Book

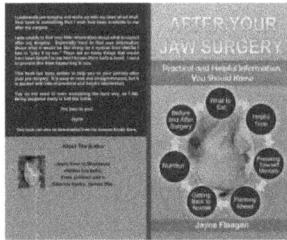

There are countless reasons that people have jaw surgery done and countless variations of the surgery.

There are also variations and different degrees of having your jaws wired shut, which is what I had done. This is also known as *maxillofacial surgery*. The gist of it is that your jaws are wired shut with metal pins and wires anchored into your jaw bones, as well as the surrounding tissues to keep your jaw from moving. These measures are taken in order to give your jaw time to heal.

Before my surgery, I started digging around for some information on what to expect after the surgery. I wanted to find out how I was going to be affected. Maybe I should have asked the oral surgeon more questions or did more research until I had a better idea of what it actually meant to have your jaws wired shut. At any rate, I was totally unprepared. I had no idea of what to expect, nor how to deal with the issues that I would face.

There are also a myriad of physiological and psychological aspects that are part of the big picture when you have jaw work done. I will cover all of these angles.

Had I known going in that I would encounter some of the things that I did along the way, I would have been more prepared. My experience would have been much more tolerable had I only known then what I know now. I think that I am a resourceful person and if it was a challenge for me to come up with answers, then other people must certainly be running into the same problem.

That is why I wrote this book. I have been there and I can help!

CHAPTER 2

On a Liquid Diet?

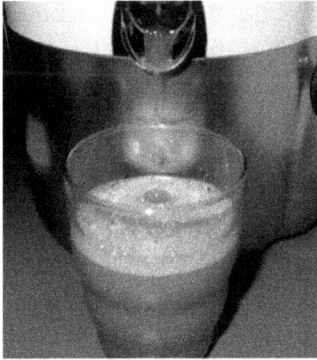

Juicing photo by leonterra, used with permission.

You will probably be on some sort of liquid or soft food diet after your surgery. The length of time will depend upon what kind of surgery you had done and when your oral surgeon gives you the go-ahead to progress to softer food, then back to your normal diet.

I was personally on a liquid diet for five weeks and five days (but who's counting?) For me, it was out of necessity because I had to have surgery to remove a cyst that was found on the left side of my jaw. After the surgery, my jaw was wired shut so it could heal and I could not eat solid foods at all. Part of the problem was that I really couldn't find much of anything about living on a liquid diet to the degree that I needed to.

I already had a good blender and a juicer with corresponding cookbooks for both of them. I thought that I was pretty well set as far as food went. What else was there to worry about? I decided that I would "play it by ear" and figure it out as I went along.

I realize now what a big mistake that was.

Even though it is temporary, living on a liquid diet involves more than a physical change in your eating habits. It truly is a drastic change in life style.

Having actually experienced having my jaws wired shut and living on a liquid diet, I know what it's like because I have "been there." You don't have to learn the hard way like I did. I will be sharing with you what I learned and what did and did not work for me.

CHAPTER 3

How Liquid is "Liquid?"

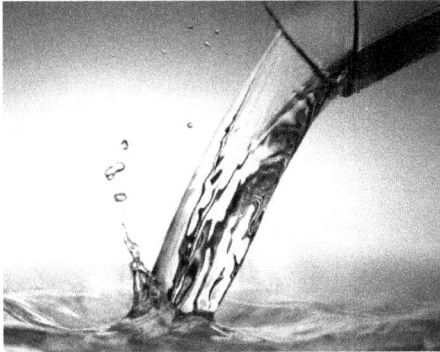

© Can Stock Photo Inc. / polichenko

Just how "liquid" your diet is depends upon your personal situation. Maybe you have had jaw surgery and don't have your jaws wired shut. Perhaps you have to deal with having rubber bands in your mouth. Maybe you will be lucky and won't have to deal with either the rubber bands or having your jaws wired, but your mouth area is sore and tender. Then you can probably have soft foods such as mashed potatoes and yogurt. That means that the thickness of your foods and how many "chunks" are in your meal is more variable and dependent upon on your taste. Your doctor should provide you with a list of foods that you'll be able to eat.

However, if your jaws are wired shut, then you are very limited! In this case, liquid is *very* liquid. If your food is too thick or is chunky, you will not even be able to get the food into your mouth, let alone be able to swallow it.

When I learned that I would be on a liquid diet, I started looking for information and recipes that I could use. What I discovered is that when people use the term "liquid diet," they may mean many different things. Many people do not understand the concept of just how liquid that recipe needs to be in some situations, such as when your jaws are wired shut.

Be careful about buying a book that says it has recipes for someone on a liquid diet. You may want to check out how the author qualifies "liquid."

Before we continue, I want to stress that this book is in no way intended to give you medical or nutritional advice. I am not an expert in either of those areas. **If you have any questions about your diet, please be sure to check with your Doctor and or a nutritionist.**

CHAPTER 4

Helpful Tools

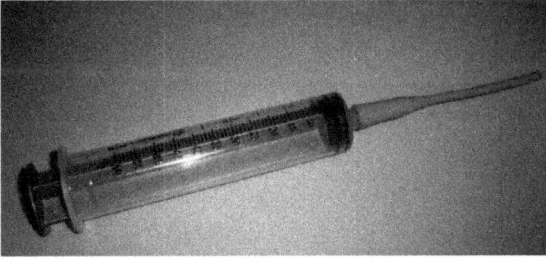

There are several handy-dandy tools that you may or may not be using while you are on your liquid diet. This will again depend upon what kind of jaw surgery you had.

Tool number one is the simple syringe. This is probably your worse-case scenario for eating. Above is a picture of the exact syringe that I ate with.

This particular syringe had flexible rubber on the front of it which you can separate from the rest of the apparatus to clean it easier. Because it is flexible in front, you can work it around in your mouth to get it to where it needs to go. You'll probably be bringing your syringe(s) home from the hospital. It may be a good idea to have a spare or two readily available when you get home as well.

One word of caution is that you'll have to keep your syringes clean. The sooner you clean them after each use, the easier it will be.

Tool number two is the pliers (which hopefully will never need to be used!)

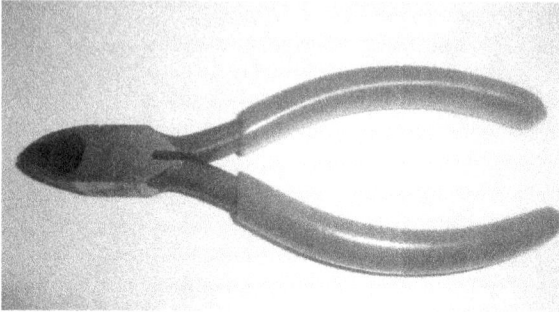

These are just a regular pair of needle-nosed pliers that the hospital sent home with me. You should receive a pair of these before you leave the hospital too. If your jaws are wired shut, you need to carry them with you at all times. You are never to use them no matter what. The only people who should use them are paramedics or emergency room staff, should they need them.

My first question was, "But what if I need to throw up?" The answer was simple: Everything went into your mouth as a liquid and that is the way it will come out if it needs to. It may come out through your nose, but it will make its way out somehow without you having to cut your wires off. If you do need to throw up, the best thing to do is to bend over and open your lips as much as possible. Thank goodness that I never had to throw up when my jaws were wired!

Tool number three is straws.

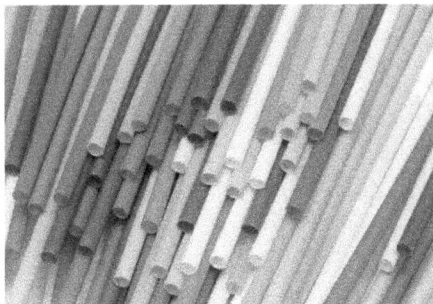

Photo by Horia Varlan, used with permission.

You may have the option of being able to use straws to eat with. You should check with your Doctor about using them. My surgeon did not want me to use a straw after my jaws were wired because sucking on a straw can put a lot of pressure on your stitches and can cause bleeding and other issues. If you are allowed to use straws, have plenty on hand and make sure that the **size of the holes** are the right ones for your needs. Also, make sure that the **ingredients in your beverage are blended well enough and thin enough to get through the straw.**

Tool number four is the pill grinder.

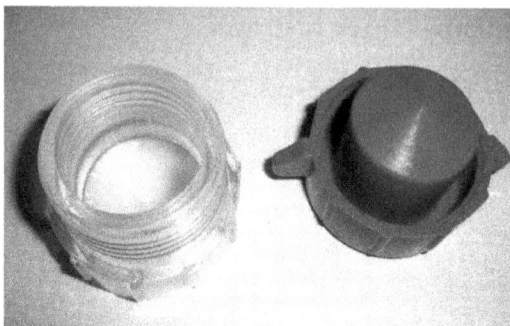

I used the above grinder for prescription medications that did not come in liquid form. In most cases, your Doctor will write your prescriptions out for the liquid form, when available. You should double-check before you leave the hospital or your Doctor's office to make sure that they are written out that way. Checking the prescription before you get to the pharmacy may save you from the hassle of getting to the pharmacy and finding out that they are in a pill form, especially if they are in a pill form that cannot be crushed. You'll save time by not having to wait while the prescription is re-filled.

You can get yourself something a bit fancier than the above pill grinder, but you probably don't need to. The grinder pictured above costs just a few dollars. You could always do what I did and ask the nurse if you could keep the one that you have been using at the hospital, as it will save you the effort of going and picking another one up.

Make sure that you grind the pills up really well. Some pills can taste very nasty if you get a chunk of one stuck in your mouth. **Also, after you grind the pill up, mix it in well with a liquid before you take it.**

Tool number five is napkins. Have them with you wherever you go because I guarantee that you will be using them! I think that's all I need to say here.

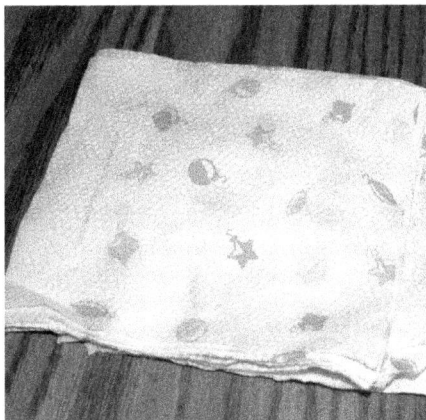

Tool number six is a good blender. I think that the very best piece of advice that I can give you regarding your liquid diet is this: **get a good blender!**

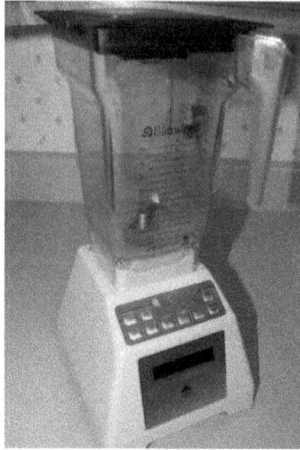

Without a powerful blender, you will end up with food chunks in your beverage that you will not be able to eat. You will also have to take the time to strain the chunks out. That strainer is just one more thing to clean. There will also be food waste because of the chunks of food that you will have to throw because you could not eat them.

As with everything else, the sooner you clean your blender, or at least rinse it out, the easier and quicker it will be to get the job done. Your blender is going to be your best friend while you are on this diet. You are going to want it to be ready to use at a moment's notice.

Even if you have to spend a little more than you normally would, a good blender, is a good investment. You can still get plenty of use out of it after you are off your liquid diet, especially if it does all of the things that my blender can do. The blender that I have can make hot soups (literally!) in just a few minutes. I do not spend money lightly, but I have not for a moment regretted spending the extra money on my blender.

You can juice versus blending your food, but there are several reasons that I don't. I find that juicing is much more work and time-consuming. Also, unless you can find some use for the pulp, it goes to the garbage and there are at least three down-sides to doing that. First, the pulp has added nutrients that you will be missing out on. Secondly, the pulp is what helps fill you up and keeps you from getting hungry. Third, there is food waste.

As you venture through your own journey, you will most likely find your own resources and tools that are most helpful to you while your jaws are wired shut. **Please share your ideas with me if you come up with any helpful hints.** I would love to hear about them! (I will include the information on how to contact me at the end of this book).

CHAPTER 5

Basic Nutrition Resources

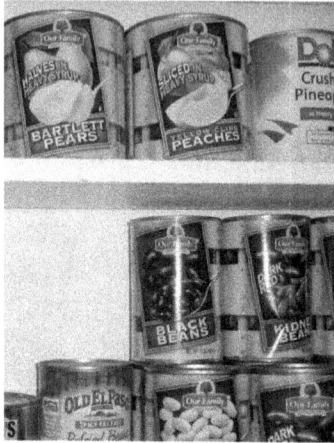

This chapter will cover information on some basic nutrients and ideas on how to use them while you are on your liquid diet.

Again, I am not intending to give nutritional advice. These are my thoughts and some of the things that worked for me personally. You need to do what works for you. Consult your doctor and/or a dietitian if you unsure if you are getting the necessary nutrients for your body. Hopefully, this chapter can at least be a starting point for some of the questions that you have. I hope it will help you figure out what aspects of this diet that you need to check into further.

1) The first thing I want to mention nutritionally is that you may want to take some liquid vitamins. You may not normally take vitamins, but there are certain nutrients that you may find harder to get into your body while you are on this diet.

The two liquid vitamins that I took on a regular basis while my jaws were wired shut were a multi-vitamin and vitamin D. I always take extra vitamin D because the last few years I have heard so much about how our bodies need much more vitamin D than we give them – especially when you live in Minnesota like I do and don't get sun for a vast majority of the year!

2) It's a good idea to try out some recipes before you begin your diet. Find some that you like and have them readily available. There will be times when you will want to eat something right away or when you are tired of store-bought shakes. Save yourself some time and frustration. Know exactly where your recipes are so that you don't have to go searching for them. You may want to put them on a computer program. It can be so much easier to organize and find them this way.

3) Make sure that you have the groceries that you need in order to make your selected recipes. If you are missing one or two ingredients, it's usually not a bit deal, as long as you have most of what you need.

As I mentioned, I began my liquid diet "playing it by ear" just a tad too much. **I quickly realized that I needed to do some planning**.

A few times I found myself just throwing whatever I could find in the refrigerator into the blender and hoped for the best. Most of the time, I really think it was the *worst*! There were actually several times that my concoction tasted so bad that I could not force myself drink it.

4) Another really nice thing to do for yourself is to have the food that you will be using washed and cut up so that it is ready to go when you are. Taking the time to get the food ready to go into the blender can be torture when you are starving and need to eat something right away. You may also be in pain after surgery, so you want to make it as easy on yourself as possible. Don't hesitate to ask those around you for help, with either getting your food ready or preparing your food, especially the days immediately following your surgery.

5) Meal replacement shakes are one of the options for getting something quick and easy into your system. These shakes are beverages designed to give you the basic nutrients that you would get if you ate a well-balanced meal. They can be purchased in powder, liquid or ready-to-drink form. You can purchase them in single serving size or larger-sized containers. I've seen a variety of flavors, depending on the brand. They always taste better cold, so don't forget to put them in the refrigerator or bring a cooler with you if you are traveling. **You should always have some of these in the ready-to-go form for certain situations**.

I spent some time researching meal replacement shakes because I did not want to put a bunch of junk in my body. What I finally decided about the meal replacement shakes is that they all have their own pros and cons.

Below is the nutrition label from one of these products. You can see that it has saturated fat, (which is said to be one of the "bad" fats) and quite a bit of sugar, but it has also has many good nutrients.

Nutrition Facts		
Serving Size 1 Packet (36 g)		
Servings Per Container 1		
Amount Per Serving		WITH 1 Cup Fat-Free Milk Vit A&D Added
Calories	130	220
Calories from Fat	5	5
		% Daily Value**
Total Fat 0.5g*	1%	1%
Sat. Fat 0g	1%	2%
Trans Fat 0g		
Cholesterol <5mg	1%	3%
Sodium 90mg	4%	8%
Potassium 320mg	9%	20%
Total Carb. 27g	9%	13%
Dietary Fiber <1g	4%	4%
Sugars 19g		
Protein 5g	10%	25%

If you want to totally control what you put in your body and you are on a liquid diet for nutrition purposes or weight loss, maybe these meal replacement drinks are not what you will want to use. However, if you are in a pinch and have no other options, they can be a lifesaver! Just a note: they are a bit pricey.

6) People drink **protein supplements** for different reasons. Body builders often use them to build muscle. I have used protein supplements off and on because I often don't get enough protein in my diet, since I do not eat very much meat.

You can get protein from other sources besides meat, of course. I consumed a lot of peanut and beans while I was on my liquid diet because they are two good sources of protein.

I spent many hours researching protein supplements too. I put together a little synopsis to give you the bare facts, as I understand them. Here we go:

Protein is known as the building blocks of muscle since it aids in the building, repair and maintenance of lean muscle tissue. Our body is not able to make some of the amino acids that protein supplements can provide us with.

A high protein diet will help to reduce hunger pangs throughout the day and suppress sweet cravings. This is important when you are on a liquid diet.

The three main kinds of protein supplements are whey, egg and casein. Each type of protein has its own pros and cons.

Casein protein is derived from cow's milk and is about 92 percent protein by weight. Because it is a slow-digesting protein, it may work well for a pre-bedtime shake to help you sleep better.

Egg protein is often derived from egg whites, so the cholesterol content is much less than whole eggs. If you are lactose intolerant or have severe milk allergies, this may be the way to go. A less expensive option is to just eat egg whites.

Whey is derived from cow's milk; it makes up about 20 percent of milk protein. Whey protein is a fast-absorbing protein source that hits your system within 20 to 40 minutes after you eat it.

There are two main types of whey protein: concentrates and isolates. Concentrate formulas of whey protein contain less protein and more lactose by weight. Isolates contain a higher level of protein and lower levels of fat or cholesterol.

If you need the added nutrition that either meal replacement shakes or protein products can provide, in order to aid you in your healing process, you may want to look into using some of them. If you do decide to use them, choose the ones that work for your needs.

CHAPTER 6

Preparing Yourself Mentally

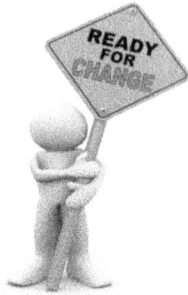

© Can Stock Photo Inc. / nasir1164

In this chapter, I am going to let you know about some things that you most likely will not be able to do if your jaws are wired shut. I am sorry to be "Debby Downer," but I think that the more you know, the more you can prepare yourself mentally for different situations that may arise. However, I will also give you some tips that will help you cope with these issues…

Licking your lips will not be an option, so you may want to have some kind of lip balm with you at all times. I don't believe it was just my imagination that my lips were extra dry after my surgery. It was torture to not have something readily available to put on my lips to moisten them.

Cleaning your teeth properly will have to be put on the back burner for a while. Brushing and/or flossing your teeth as well as you like will not be possible. Make sure that you ask your doctor before you go home how he wants you to keep your mouth and teeth clean. It's important not to get lax with this because it will help prevent infection and other issues inside your mouth. **Actually, it will be necessary to clean your teeth more often than you did before your surgery**. This is because you will be eating more often and you need to clean your mouth and teeth as soon as you can each time after eating.

I used a **child's soft tooth brush while my jaws were wired.** It worked much better than an adult-sized toothbrush because I was able to reach some of my back teeth a little easier and it treated my mouth more gently. **Then I rinsed my mouth out with a solution of one teaspoon of salt in a warm cup of water.**

Ask your doctor if you can use a **Water-Pik** and which setting you can use it on, if it has different options. (I wish that I had thought of a Water Pik earlier)!

Even if you do your best to keep your mouth clean, your teeth are still probably going to feel gritty. My teeth certainly did. I was sure that my teeth were going to be in really bad shape by the time I could brush them properly again. However, when I had my teeth cleaned a couple of months after having had the wires taken out, the Dentist said that my teeth looked great. All you can do is your best!

One of the other benefits of keeping your mouth clean is that it will be easier to talk. Your words will come out much clearer and people will understand you better. (Seriously).

Speaking of talking, my advice is that you should try to do as little of it as possible. Of course sometimes you will need to talk. Your words won't come out perfectly clear, but most of the time you can make yourself understood. However, yelling is another matter. Since talking can be tough, you can bet that yelling to someone is not going to be an option. I remember trying to yell downstairs to my son or holler something to my husband in the back yard. Nothing came out but an odd, guttural sound. If you need someone's attention, you are just going to have to go to that person.

(I will cover the topic of talking a bit more in another chapter).

Coughing, sneezing and yawning are all going to be tough with your jaws wired shut. In fact, sneezing can be downright painful. I think that I just kind of "braced myself and went with it!" (No, you cannot actually blow your brains out by sneezing hard even though it might feel like you did sometimes).

Smiling normally gets quite interesting results. Don't plan on any family photos while your teeth are wired, unless you don't plan on smiling. No matter how hard you try, you probably are not going to get a "full" smile out and you won't look like you normally would.

You obviously won't be able to eat the same meal as everyone else. In fact, being in the same room while everyone else is eating their meal may be hard on you. If it does not bother you, good for you! However, if it is too hard on you, don't feel badly if you need to eat at a different time and/or place than the rest of your family.

I remember one night in particular, my husband made tuna fish sandwiches for supper. A few weeks before that night, I would never have imagined that tuna fish could smell so good! He was also eating fresh tomatoes and cucumbers from the garden, which I look forward to all winter long. (He did try to be kind and tell me they tasted terrible. However, I knew that he was lying because of the way he was drooling as he ate them).

Kissing - What can I say? You'll have to find out for yourself about this one. During my surgery, the Doctor hit a nerve in the area where the cyst was removed. I was advised before surgery that it would be hard *not* to nick that nerve because the cyst was so large.

This nick affected all of my bottom lip as well as most of my chin and the left side of my face. As I write this, it has been five months since the surgery and it still feels as though I have a permanent Novocain drip in that part of my face. It's very sensitive and feels as though it is swollen. It may or may not be permanent. I am still waiting to see.

Getting back to exercise is another thing that you need to talk to your Doctor about. You should find out what kind of exercises you can do and how long you should wait before you start them. If your Doctor gives you the "okay" for things such as walking or riding a bicycle, you should try to do it.

I had been swimming a mile several times a week and putting in four to five miles on the elliptical several days a week before my surgery. I certainly was not up to any of that for quite some time after the surgery! Hopefully, we all know the benefits of exercising, so the only other thing that I am going to add here is to try and get the proper nutrients every day because that will help keep up your energy level and you will be more motivated to exercise.

Smoking: I have never smoked, so this is one thing that I never had to worry about. If you do smoke, and you know that you will be having your jaws wired, this might be a good time to quit! There are many products on the market to help you with this. At any rate, you should probably decide as soon as possible how you are going to deal with this issue. You're going to have to quit smoking while you're in the hospital at least. Again, talk to your Doctor; he may prescribe something to help you with it.

Basically, many of the things that you take for granted will become issues when your jaws are wired shut. How big those issues become is

mostly going to be determined by how well you handle them. Just keep reminding yourself that your situation is only temporary. For whatever reason you had the work done on your jaw, it's a good enough reason to put up with some temporary problems.

CHAPTER 7

The Day Before Surgery: Fill 'er up?

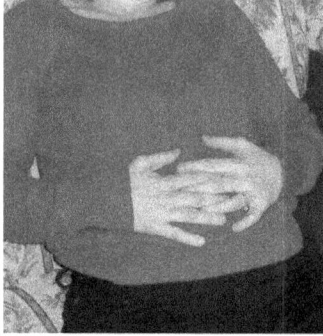

As is typical before most surgeries or when you have to go in for blood work, I was told not to eat at least eight hours before the surgery.

The evening before surgery, I went out to eat pasta with my husband and my sister. I knew I wouldn't have a "real" meal for who knows how long so I ate *way* more than I normally would have. I finished off the entire dish, practically licking the plate. Typically, I would have taken a large portion of the meal home in a doggy bag and had two more meals out of that one entrée.

I certainly didn't give my stomach time to register how full it was as I continued to eat. As is typical with a salty meal, I was really thirsty afterwards. However, since I was such a pig and had eaten so much food, I did not have any more room in my stomach for water. Thus, I went to bed uncomfortably full and thirsty. If I had to do it all over again, I would certainly not "stock up" the night before. It simply was not worth it!

Getting back to the topic of drinking water, you may need to remind yourself to drink more water while you are on this diet. It will probably feel as though you are already getting enough liquids because, after all, everything that you are eating is in liquid form. **However, you still need to make sure that you drink plenty of plain water on a regular basis.**

Sometimes when you think you are hungry, your body is just craving water. Drinking some water can either alleviate or temporarily take care of your hunger pangs.

What you do or do not eat the night before your surgery is obviously up to you. I know that if I had to do it all over again, I think that I would be more focused on getting more liquids in me versus eating such a big meal!

CHAPTER 8

Surgery Day

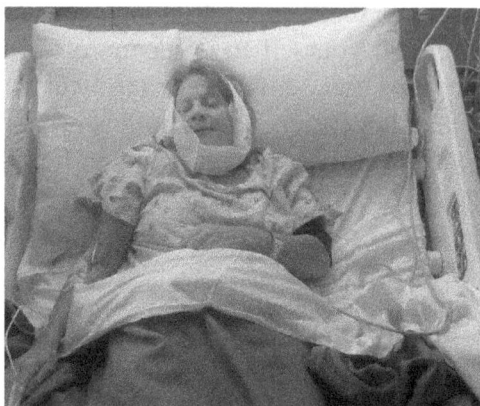

By the time surgery day rolled around, I was just looking forward to getting it over and done with.

The morning of surgery, I was allowed to drink clear liquids up to two hours before the procedure. Clear liquids include such things as water, broth, plain gelatin, clear sodas and fruit juices without any pulp – and thank goodness, coffee! I would have had a serious caffeine withdrawal had I not been able to have my cup of Joe. (You can have clear liquids because they are easily digested and leave no residue in your intestinal tract).

Our report time for surgery was 9:30 a.m., so I quit drinking liquids at 7:30 that morning. We did not get into surgery for another three hours. By that time, I was really thirsty. When the nurse tried to put the needle into my arm for the IV, my vein "blew up". (A "blown vein" is when the needle punctures not only the vein, but another spot as well). My arm swelled up a bit where the needle had gone in, but otherwise it was no big deal.

The nurse said that if I had more water in my system, that probably would not have happened. (She may actually have done a poor job with the needle insertion and was too embarrassed to say so). Just to be on the safe side, though, drinking plenty of water while you can is almost always a good option.

Regarding surgery, everyone's situation is different, depending upon what you are having done and many other factors. Therefore, I am not going to go into details about what to expect immediately after surgery and the days and weeks following. I can only tell you a bit about my experiences and try to give you some general tips that you will be able to use.

During the surgery, the sedation had me completely "out." I learned later that besides the sedation, I was also given an amnesia drug so that I would not remember anything, so I actually don't even remember getting sedated.

During my surgery, the Doctor removed two teeth on top of the cyst in order to get to the cyst directly. He then removed the cyst and a bone graph was placed in part of the area where the cyst had been. The graph was placed there for new bone growth to have something to latch on to. The idea is that eventually my jaw bone will grow back where the cyst had replaced it.

I was told that surgery could take between one and four hours, depending on what they "found when they got in there." Later, my husband told me that the surgery lasted just a little over an hour and twenty minutes. (He times almost everything to the minute. This included our wedding and he informed me not too long after leaving the church that day exactly how long the ceremony was).

My scenarios could have turned out much worse, so I was happy with the outcome. For one thing, the surgeon was able to go through the inside of my mouth to get to the cyst, versus cutting on the outside of my face. I was also happy that I did not need to have any metal plates put in my mouth, which was also a possibility.

However, they did indeed wire my jaws shut because of the extensive bone loss in the jaw area. The surgeon wanted to give the bone graph some time to "toughen up" and wiring my jaws shut would help lessen the chances of my jaw getting broke.

I cannot show you what it looked like inside my mouth, but it felt as though there were wires everywhere! However, I *can* show you what it looked like on the outside, as you can see in the picture below.

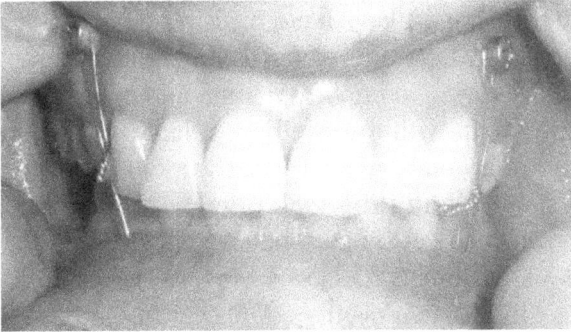

Two screws were put into my upper gums and two were put into my lower gums to help "anchor" things in. (This picture was actually taken a few weeks after surgery).

Probably one of the worst things about having jaw surgery, especially if your jaws get wired shut, is waking up from surgery and not being able to talk. It's hard to prepare yourself for something like that. You'll realize quickly that your jaws will tire easily, which is why I suggested earlier in the book that you probably should talk as little as possible.

As time passes, people will most likely be able to understand most of what you are saying. You may have to figure out how to move your tongue and mouth to get your words out clearer. Those closest to you may get used to your new way of speaking pretty quickly. Especially for the first few days after surgery, you may want to have pen and paper handy so that you can write things down when you need to.

You will most likely have bruising and swelling in your face after surgery. I was given the contraption (I am wearing it in the picture under this chapter title) to help with the swelling. It had ice in in and it wrapped around my jaw. What worked better for me was a **very long tube sock filled with ice**. The sock was easier to get snug around my face so that the ice had more impact. Also, it stayed on better. You won't look like a beauty contestant in either one, so you may as well use whatever works the best!

Often, the swelling will actually get worse after a couple of days. You will want to keep up on the ice packs for relief. **Sleeping with your head raised at night when you sleep will help with the swelling.**

You will probably be given at least a couple of medications while you are in the hospital and probably prescriptions for re-fills before you leave the hospital. I'm sure that at least one of them will be a pain medication. **A notebook is a good way to keep track of what time you took each medication. You will probably need to alternate pain medications, so writing things down will keep you on track.**

What's really important is to keep on top of your medications **so that you can keep on top of the pain**. I made the mistake several times of holding off on my medications too long because I didn't feel "too bad." However, what often happens when you do start hurting worse, is that the pain can hit you pretty hard. At that point, you will have a harder time getting your pain to abate than if you had taken you medications on time.

Also, remember not to take your pain medications on an empty stomach! Read the label on your medication and take them with food as directed. Otherwise, you could experience stomach problems as a side effect.

So what about eating at this point? Right up until surgery all I could think about was eating and getting something to drink. After surgery, it was the last thing on my mind until later that evening when I could not ignore the growling in my stomach any longer.

Below is a copy of my menu for the day. Yum yum!

CLEAR LIQUID DIET

Juice ● (4-ounce Cup)
Apple, Cranberry or Grape

Broth
Vegetable, Chicken or Beef

Other
Coffee, Decaf Coffee
Hot Tea (Black, Green or Herbal)
Iced Tea (Regular and Decaf)
Kool-Aid,* Lemonade, Gatorade*

The Finishing Touch
Fruit Ice - Lemon or Raspberry ●, *Gelatin ●
*Popsicles

*Available in Sugar Free

I decided to go with the cranberry juice for my evening "meal." My throat was quite sore, so it took me a couple of hours to drink a four ounce container of juice. My tool at that time was the syringe. You probably know how that works. First you "suck" the food up with the syringe, then you push on the back of the syringe to get the food into your mouth. It takes time and effort, so eating is not going to be a speedy endeavor at this point.

Using the syringe was actually a little easier for me than it might be for some people. I had two missing molars in the back of my mouth so once I got the syringe "around the corner," I actually had a pocket of sorts to squeeze the food into. Otherwise, your only other choice of insertion may be the thin gap in the front of your mouth where your upper teeth may "overhang" your lower teeth a bit.

That night in the hospital, I could not sleep for various reasons, so I thought that eating something might help. However, the kitchen was closed and the nurse said that the only thing that he could bring me was some ice cream. I waited until the ice cream melted and tried to eat that, but it was still too thick, so I gave up.

While you are in the hospital, even if you are not hungry at the time, you may want to order something from the kitchen before is closes. That way, you will have something to eat should you choose to do so later in the evening.

Hopefully, during your hospital stay you will have someone with you most of the time. My husband had to leave right after my surgery. I was blessed to have my sister Kathy with me, who waited on me hand and foot. I was so thankful that she was there, because the nursing staff was almost non-existent.

One of the things that surprised me after surgery was the number of machines hooked up to me. The first nurse that I had in the hospital told me to make sure that I buzzed her when I needed to go to the bathroom. She helped me walk to the bathroom and unplug and re-plug the machines back in. However, the night nurse that was supposed to attend to me said that I was OK to do those things on my own. I accepted that from him, but I really should not have. It was still hard to get to the bathroom on my own. Once I unplugged the machines, I couldn't figure out where to plug them back in. (My sister had gone home for the night, thinking that I would basically be sleeping all night).

During your hospital stay you should expect the hospital staff to do their job. Don't take it upon yourself to do things that you should not be doing yet and are not trained to do!

You don't want to fall or do something that could put you right back in the surgery room.

CHAPTER 9

"Eating" the Days Following Surgery

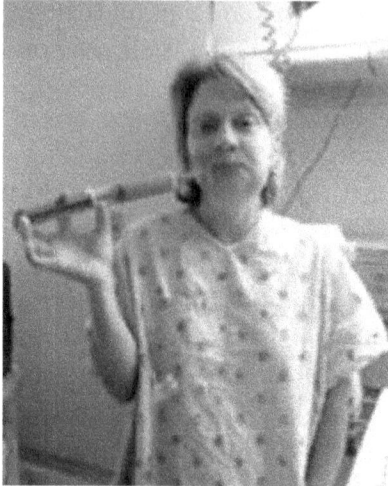

If you are a coffee drinker, you may be "siphoning" your coffee in the next morning, as I had to do.

I was encouraged to use a cup if possible to drink in the small gap between my top and bottom front teeth. **It helps to remember a couple of things when eating or drinking. The first is that liquids have to be very thin in consistency. The second thing is that you need to drink slowly and in very small sips**. If your drink is too thick or if you try and drink it too fast, you may make a mess of yourself and find it all over your shirt.

The day after surgery, I ordered pureed potato soup, pureed lasagna and a thin milkshake for lunch. They were all actually edible, even though drinking my lasagna was rather odd.

It took me quite some time to eat enough to where I felt comfortably satiated.

Something I quickly figured out was that if you get food on the outside of the syringe, it helps to wipe it off before you try and eat any more. If you don't, you will probably find your food everywhere else but in your mouth, as I did.

That afternoon in the hospital, the nutritionist came in to offer some suggestions for what to eat in the upcoming weeks. She gave me two small booklets. One of the booklets was called "Nutritious and Flavorful Blended Meals". The idea behind the recipes in this book was that you make your meals as you normally would, then simply add liquid to them and puree them in the blender. You could have a tuna fish sandwich, a cheeseburger, or lasagna as I did – just in liquid form.

I did plan on trying some of the recipes in the book along the way. But, I knew that I would never try some of the others, such as the "fish burger" recipe. There was absolutely no way that I would be siphoning a liquid fish recipe into *this* mouth!

Before you check out of the hospital, there are several things that you may want to have the answer to before you leave.

If your surgery is done out of town, make sure that you have a Dentist or Oral Surgeon that you can see if you have issues once you get back home. One of the problems that I encountered after my surgery was that some wires had come loose and they were poking on the inside of my mouth. If something like that happens to you, will want to have someone close to where you live available to do what they can to help.

Another problem I had was that two of the screws in my mouth were rubbing the inside of my cheeks and getting caught on my lips almost every time I opened my mouth. To alleviate this problem, I picked up some dental wax to put over the screws to ease the chafing. It wasn't a perfect solution, but it felt much better.

Two things that I learned about using the dental wax:

1) Make sure that you get some before you leave the hospital

2) You may not want to leave it in overnight. When I left the wax in my mouth overnight, it dislodged and went everywhere. It's very hard to retrieve pieces of wax stuck all over the inside of your mouth when you have nothing to try and reach it but your tongue! At any rate, if you don't get some dental wax from the hospital before you leave, you should ask someone to get some for you.

Before you leave the hospital, visit with your Doctor about when it is safe to go back to work. Find out if you have any work restrictions. Make sure that he/she knows what you do for a living, so that you can get a better time frame for when you can go back to doing your normal job if you are temporarily restricted from it. I was working with small children when I had my surgery. However, the six weeks that my jaws were wired and for a few weeks after, I was given a "Doctor's note" restricting me from working directly with children. (The oral surgeon said that there are lots of people who actually get their jaws broken by children, such as when they are playing with them or even just holding a child on their lab and the child suddenly jerks his/her head up and hits you in the jaw).

Make sure that you keep your work supervisor informed of your restrictions. **It is in your best interests to follow doctor's orders and not push yourself to do things that you are not ready for yet.**

Since you will have been under anesthesia, you should not be driving for at least 48 hours after your surgery. Most likely, you won't be released from the hospital unless you have a driver to take you home, which hopefully won't be an issue.

Any time that you are on certain medications, you should not be driving. **Make sure that you know which medications to avoid if you need to drive. If you are going back to work after surgery and are still on certain medications, you may want to**

think about car-pooling or having someone drive you to work for a while.

Your Doctor should give you other instructions about what you can and cannot do. Avoiding heavy lifting and strenuous exercise were two of my directives. **If you have questions about anything, ask, ask, ask! No question is too trivial.**

Back to the food topic...**before you leave the hospital, have food readily available in a form that you can eat!**

That evening (after having left the hospital in the afternoon), we were to go to my sister's house for dinner. I had not even planned that far ahead. So while my sister was helping me check out and get my medications at the hospital, my husband was running around trying to round up some liquid meal replacements for me.

For dinner, I drank a container of vanilla *Boost* while my husband and other three family members were eating homemade margarita pizza, which had fresh tomatoes and basil on it. It smelled so good... That was my first real "taste" of feeling deprived and it would not be my last one.

CHAPTER 10

Keeping a Positive Attitude

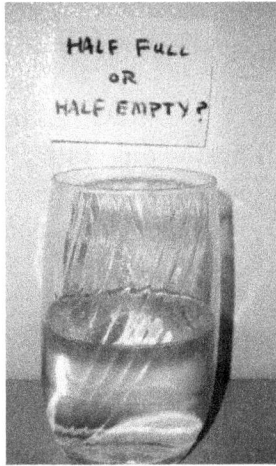

We all get frustrated from time to time and have "bad days." I put the words "bad days" in parentheses because each of us has more control over those days than we probably realize. The control we have – and yes, you have heard it before – is how we react to the things that happen to us. Sometimes, if we think back, we may even have had some control over whether or not the "bad thing" even had to happen in the first place.

I remember one morning when I was getting particularly frustrated. I had been trying to syringe my breakfast in. The syringe came apart at least two times that morning and the food in it squirted everywhere. I could hear my Mother in my head telling me to slow down and stop trying to rush everything. She was right; I know that if I had not been trying to rush things so much that morning, the syringe would not have popped apart, I would not have gotten frustrated and I would have been more positive on the way to work that day. So again, sometimes we have more control than we think.

I am sorry to say that you will have your moments like this too. **About the only thing that you can do is to move on, learn from the experience, and hope that your outcome will be better the next time**.

Some days people might say things to you such as, "I should get my jaws wired shut. I bet I could lose a lot of weight!" A natural instinct might be to think what an insensitive jerk that person is being. Or, you can take the comment as it was meant to be – just an innocent remark from that person saying that he/she needs to lose some weight.

There are other things that you can do to help keep a positive attitude.

For instance, you can **treat yourself now and then to some tasty foods**! You don't want to feel deprived the entire time that you are on this diet. I didn't have any fun foods, such as a runny ice cream shake the whole time that my jaws were wired because I wanted to eat as nutritiously as possible the whole time. However, it seems that the minute my jaws were "unwired," I have been making up for it ever since. If you are on a liquid diet to lose weight, you may end up gaining more weight in the end by over-compensating later to make up for having felt deprived while you are on the diet.

You can treat yourself in other "non-food" ways also. Try a relaxing bath, a good book or shopping, if that's what you enjoy. It won't make up for the food that you cannot have, but treating yourself a little more than you normally do may help compensate somehow.

Basically, you can choose to realize that the situation is "what it is," keep reminding yourself that it's only temporary and make the best of it (and also impress everyone around you by how well you are handling things). Or, you can choose to whine about it and make everyone else's life miserable too.

It's your decision, but choose wisely!

CHAPTER 11

Getting a Balanced Diet and Not Going Hungry

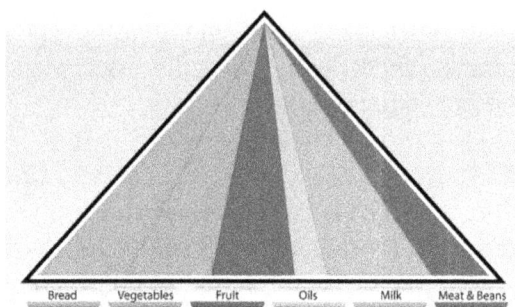

© Can Stock Photo Inc. / cteconsulting

I am assuming that you care about your health, so while you are on your liquid diet, you will want to get the proper nutrients. You also want to make sure that you get enough of the right nutrients into your system to help keep you feeling full, so that you don't feel hungry all the time.

When I first started eating with my jaws wired, I decided that the easiest way for me to get the proper nutrients would be to make my food how I normally do. I would then run them through the blender in order to get it into my system, just as the book from the hospital suggested.

This lasted about two days. I decided it was just not for me.

There is a reason they call certain foods casseroles, some are called salads, some are called sandwiches, etc. It's because they are meant to be eaten a certain way. For instance, a sandwich is usually some meat and maybe a few other ingredients eaten between two slices of bread. A casserole is several different ingredients layered together a certain way and salads are made up of different ingredients tossed together. An important factor here is that the ingredients are "separate" enough so that you can taste each ingredient and feel the texture of the ingredients somewhat independently of the others.

One can even make a definite distinction between stews, soups and purees. I tend to think of stews as ingredients cooked together but the ingredients are of different textures, sizes and shapes. A soup, on the other hand, is composed of different ingredients that are mixed together, but with fewer variations in texture and food chunks than you would find in a stew. The ingredients in a puree, meanwhile, are completely blended together so that there is only one over-all taste and texture.

What I decided while I was on my "no-chew" diet, was that most of my meals were basically going to be recipes for pureed soups - how they were designed to be eaten. I knew that I would need to get a variety of nutrients in recipes to try and cover the food groups, but at least there was a better chance that they would be more appealing to me. You need to do whatever works for you.

One of the most important things to remember to do is to eat often. Since you are drinking your meal, you are going to feel hungry sooner than if you had eaten a meal of solid food. Your liquid meal is in a more digestible form, so your body is going to process it faster. Even if the food started out as a solid, you will still get hungry sooner.

Maybe part of the equation is psychological because you didn't cut up and chew your food as you normally do. Whatever factors are involved, eating more often will help with this issue. Going overboard in one sitting and trying to "stock up" on calories doesn't seem to work either. You will just feel bloated and uncomfortable. That was my experience, at least.

You are also going to feel tired and sluggish if you aren't eating properly and it is going to be difficult to make it through your day. Some days after work, I would literally crawl into the house and drag myself over to the couch. I stayed there the rest of the evening until I finally dragged myself to bed. It's frustrating, especially if there are things that you need to get done.

Another suggestion I have for you is to keep a detailed food log. Write down exactly what and how much you eat as soon as you eat it, so that you don't forget. Include your water intake on the log. When you are eating many of the same foods on a regular basis, you may forget what you put in your stomach last and at what time you did so. **Keeping a food log will help you keep track of both your food and water intake and help ensure that you are getting enough of both.**

One way to alleviate hunger pains is to make your meals more satisfying and filling. Fiber, protein and fat are some really critical ingredients to get in your smoothies to help give you that sense of fullness.

A **protein supplement may be your surest and easiest way to get more protein.** Some other good sources of protein are **peanut butter** and **Greek yogurt** (not low-fat). Good sources of fiber are **flaxseed, wheat germ oat bran and chia seeds** (all ground of course). Foods like bananas are always good "fillers".

Sometimes I put a little **olive oil** in my drinks. **Remember that our bodies need "good oils" and they have the added benefit of helping us fill more satiated at the same time.**

Below are a couple of good-tasting, filling shakes that I made numerous times. (I varied my shakes as much as possible by rotating ingredients and you can do the same. You don't ever have to follow most recipes exactly to get a good result).

Peanut Butter Smoothie

1 cup almond or soy milk
1 ripe banana
2-3 pitted dates (for sweetener, or maple syrup to
taste)
2 tbsp. peanut butter (or other nut or seed butters)
1/4 to 1/2 cup oats
1 tbsp. chia seeds

Super foods Smoothie:

1 cup almond or soy milk
1 ripe banana
1 cup frozen fruit (usually berries)
2 tbsp. chia seeds
2 tbsp. milled flax seeds
2-5 cups spinach or shredded kale
1 scoop protein powder (optional)

For both recipes, mix thoroughly in the blender of
course!

The infamous Dr. Oz says that adding plain gelatin
to your diet gives you lots of extra nutrients and
helps you feel fuller so that you sleep better. My
sister suggested this, but I forgot to try it.

**Speaking of sleep, a good time to have a more
filling shake is before you go to bed.** I remember
getting up in the middle of night being very hungry
at times. I didn't want to put ice cubes in the
blender in the middle of the night and wake up the

whole house. I also didn't feel like having strained vegetable soup at that time in the morning either.

At the very least, try not to go to bed already hungry. If you are like me, you won't be able to sleep well. Also, it will save you from having to drag yourself out of bed to find food, then having to brush your teeth again.

If you are at all concerned about gaining weight while you are on your liquid diet, I wouldn't be. I think that would be very hard to do. It's more important that you get the right nutrients and make sure that you are not depriving yourself either psychologically or physically.

If you take care of yourself, this whole experience will be so much more tolerable for you.

CHAPTER 12

Recipes

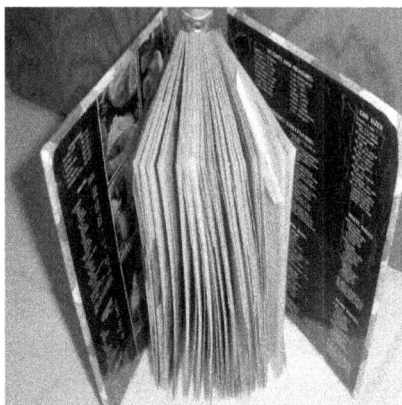

In this chapter I have included several more recipes. This first recipe is one that taught me a lesson right away.

Veggie Cocktail

½ cup plain nonfat yogurt
½ cup peeled cucumber
¼ cup fresh broccoli
¾ cup frozen peas
1/3 tsp garlic powder
1//4 – 1/2 cup ice cubes

This was a recipe that I would have really liked - if I had left out the peas. Don't ever feel as though you need to make a recipe exactly as it is. If there is an ingredient in the recipe that you don't like, leave it out. Otherwise, it will ruin the whole "dining" experience for you and you may not be able to make yourself drink it.

Here's another recipe:

Zucchini Soup

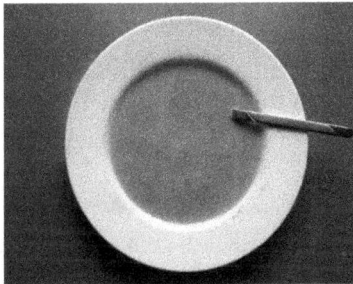

Soup photo by Wolfgang, used with permission.

Ingredients:

2 cups (480 ml) chicken broth
1/2 cup (120 ml) half and half, heavy cream, or milk
1 teaspoon lemon juice
1 medium zucchini, chopped
1 medium carrot, halved
1/2 celery stalk
1 teaspoon diced green bell pepper
1/2 potato, scrubbed, baked
Salt and pepper

Directions: Put all of the Ingredients in the blender and mix very well. Add salt and pepper to taste and warm up on the stove or in the microwave after it is blended.

This soup had a good flavor. I added more pepper and some other spices because I like things "zippy," which really helps liven things up when you are only eating soups every day.

When I made soups, I always made extra and I made at least two kinds so that I could rotate them out. That way I wasn't eating the same soup several meals in a row.

I almost always use dried beans in my soup recipes. They are dirt cheap and you can control the amount of salt that goes into your recipes. If you have never done this, you just soak the beans overnight, then cook them the next day until they are tender, at which point they are ready to go into your recipe. If you don't want to bother with this, there are many different kinds of beans readily available in cans. Maybe you could take this "opportunity" and try out some different kinds of beans that you have never eaten before!

A couple of other good things about beans is that they help you feel full longer and they are a good source of protein, especially chick peas, otherwise known as garbanzo beans.

Below is a recipe using chick peas.

Chickpea and Spinach Soup (puree)

Onion to taste
Garlic to taste
2-3 cups chicken or vegetable broth
½ green pepper
3 cups fresh spinach
4 cups cooked chick peas
1 tsp. cumin
1 tsp. curry powder
Salt & pepper to taste

Sauté the onion, garlic and pepper in some olive oil. Add everything together in your blender and warm up once the ingredients are well-blended.

As I mentioned earlier, if you have a blender that makes the soup, including heating it up, your soup will be ready to go straight out of the blender! Here are a few **fruit smoothie recipes** that you may want to try:

Peach Smoothie

Almond milk
cut up fresh peaches
honey, to taste
plain Greek yogurt
a banana
fresh spinach
whey protein powder
ice cubes

Fresh Fruit Smoothie

(talk about getting your fruits in for the day!)
2 cups grapes
1 cup strawberries
1 cup watermelon
1/2 cup cantaloupe
1/2 cup pineapple
1/2 peeled banana
1 1/2 cups ice

Banana Smoothie

1/2 cup orange juice
1 tsp. vanilla
honey, to taste
2 peeled bananas
3 cups ice

If you put the ice cubes in the bottom of the blender along with some liquid (milk in this case), they will crush up better.

You can actually make any "fruit smoothie" with just some yogurt and/or tofu, milk (any kind), your favorite fruit and a sweetener if you choose. I usually use either honey or agave syrup for my sweeteners.

And now for some veggie recipes…!

Tomato Carrot Juice

1 medium tomato, halved
1 carrot, cut into a few pieces
1/2 cup broccoli
ice and water at the bottom of the blender

Tomato Broccoli Juice

1 cup of any kind of grapes
3 large tomatoes
1/2 cup fresh broccoli
ice
(It's amazing what a difference the grapes make in sweetness and flavor!)

Fresh Vegetable Juice

3 large tomatoes
1/4 medium onion
1 stalk celery, cut into a few pieces
1 carrot, cut into a few pieces
ice cubes and water

You know the routine – blend it all together very well before drinking!

I did not get to fully enjoy "reaping" in our garden vegetables this year since my jaws were wired shut most of the summer. However, many of the ingredients that I used in my soups and smoothies did come from my garden. The vegetables I used the most were kale and spinach. They were readily available, fresh and organic.

When you make your blender foods, don't be afraid to add an ingredient or so that the recipe does not call for. Be careful not to overdo it, though. I went overboard with some of the garden foods, trying to make sure that they didn't go to waste and ended up ruining my meal.

Another thing that I usually added to my cold drinks was extra ice cubes because I like my cold drinks cold and they stayed cold longer. Don't add too many ice cubes, though, or you will end up with a very bland, watery beverage!

Using Herbs and a Few More Recipes

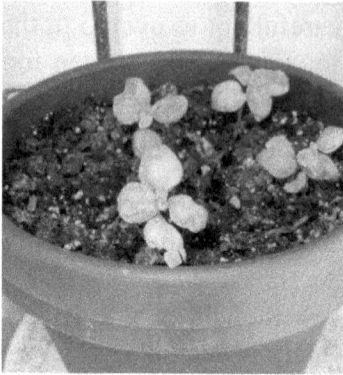

The FDA cautions people to be wary of herbal supplements, but in this instance I am referring to pure, fresh herbs here, which are usually entirely different. I don't think most people realize how many healthy benefits there are to fresh herbs. They provide both good flavor and tons of nutritional benefits!

I used to use a lot more salt in what I ate, but since I started growing my own herbs and using them, I don't miss the salt nearly as much.

Basil is by far the herb that I use the most, especially when I was on my liquid diet. I also used a lot of fun, spicy seasonings such as cumin and turmeric. An added bonus is that the soups usually come out a very pretty color, making them more appealing to the eye.

Here are a couple of soup recipes which I came up with, using plenty of herbs for seasonings. I named the first one "Green Soup" because I used almost all green vegetables. I'm sure that you could probably come up with a better name for it than that, though…

GREEN SOUP RECIPE

In olive oil, sauté onions, garlic, broccoli and green pepper. Add these to the blender with some chicken broth, cut up zucchini, curry, avocado, parsley,marjoram, oregano and red pepper seasonings.
Puree and you're done!

CHICKPEA (GARBANZO BEANS) SOUP

Sauté some onions and garlic in olive oil. Add it to the blender with about 3-4 cups of chickpeas (either from the can or soaked the night before and cooked until soft). Add some tofu in for extra protein and thickness, some bacon bits (either real or from the jar, but the "real ones are better-tasting of course)," cumin and curry powder to taste. (I used a healthy teaspoon of each of the seasonings). Put it in the blender, puree, heat up and you've got yourself a very colorful, very flavorful soup!

You will notice that there are no amounts listed for the ingredients in the above recipes. Since I "invented" these recipes, I basically put the foods into the blender jar until it reached the "full" line, without worrying too much about exact quantities of anything. Sometimes it didn't work that well, but most of the time, the soups were fine. You can try the recipes and then adapt them by adding more of what you like and less of what you don't! Be adventurous!

CHAPTER 13

Allow Yourself More Time

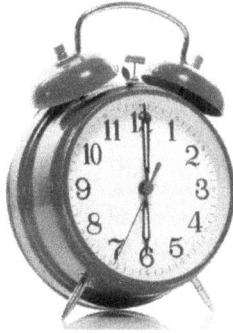

© Can Stock Photo Inc. / artjazz

It wasn't too long after coming home from the hospital, that I realized I needed more time to get ready to go places, especially in the morning. Between having to crush up my medications, clean the blender, and either syringe or slowly sip my breakfast, I found myself speeding to work to make it there on time.

A couple of things that you can do to alleviate the morning rush is either to get up a little earlier in the morning or do as much as you can the night before. I know- that sounds just like something your mother probably told you to do and she was right.

In the evening, you can crush your morning pills and have your blender food washed and cut up. If you are having a meal replacement beverage, things will go a little faster. However, if you just have one of the meal replacement beverages with nothing else added, you will probably need to eat something again sooner than you normally would need to because they are just not that filling.

Some nights I made my shakes up for the next day. It helped save some time, but in the morning, even when I re-blended them with fresh ice cubes, they weren't as good as when I made them fresh. So I went back to making them fresh in the morning. (My kids didn't care for the sound of the blender crushing up ice in the wee hours of the morning, but by then they had pretty much figured out it was best not to say anything!)

If you do some planning and prepare a bit ahead of time, you will be less stressed from the rush of trying to get somewhere on time.

CHAPTER 14

Planning Ahead For Trips

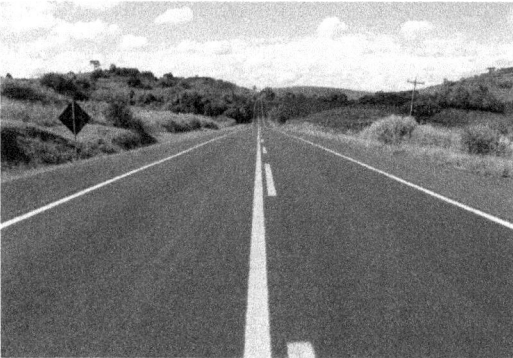

© Can Stock Photo Inc. / iDesign

I have mentioned planning ahead and being prepared at least a couple of times in this book. In this particular chapter, I am referring to when you go out of town for the day or longer.

Here's what happened to me because I did not take the time to plan further down the road…

My husband and I left our house one Saturday for a three-hour trip to a wedding. A half hour out of town, I was already hungry. I had a pretty filling smoothie early that morning, but I had *meant* to also have some soup before I left. I ran out of time because I was trying to get other things done before we left so I forgot. I also *meant* to take some extra soup with me because they filled me up longer than the meal replacement shakes did. That's what I *meant* to do.

I had all of the right clothes, a swim suit, things to read, my make-up, etc, but I really wasn't prepared when it came to my eating plan for the next two days.

Instead, I left the house with five or six of those 8-ounce bottles of ready-made supplement drinks. They were all the same brand and all chocolate.

I was so hungry the entire weekend and I had a splitting headache from not getting enough food in me. By the end of those two days it almost made me physically ill to even look at the shakes that I had brought with me because I was so tired of them.

I chose to skip the reception after the wedding because I did not want to be around all of that food that I could not eat. Instead, I went back to the hotel room and rested for awhile before the dance. My jaws were really hurting and I felt really exhausted. Before the wedding, I had spent several hours explaining to everyone why my jaws were wired shut, which of course made them hurt worse. Going back to the hotel and resting was definitely a good decision for me.

Later that evening at the dance, I found myself explaining to even more people about my situation. It wasn't too long before my jaws and head were absolutely throbbing again. I finally had my husband take me back to the hotel, because by that time I was in really bad shape.

The next day at the hotel was not any better. Below is a picture of my two-course breakfast. It's a glass of watered-down orange juice and a cup of coffee.

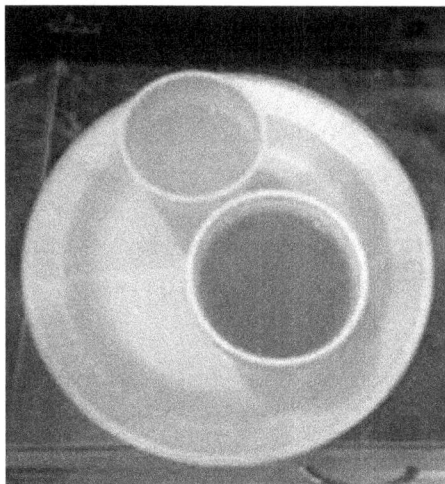

I tried to mix a packet of oatmeal with lots of water, but the flakes were too big to make it past the entry point to get into my mouth.

When we headed back home that weekend, I found myself dreaming about having a bowl of pureed spinach soup that I had in the refrigerator. Before this outing, I would never have imagined that I would be eagerly anticipating such a weird thing.

Unless you want to be miserably hungry like I was all weekend, plan ahead and bring something more "substantial" to eat than a six-pack of chocolate something-or-other.

That weekend, I had wanted to visit with people and not miss out on anything. I also didn't want to offend anyone, so I just plain over-did it. If I had to do it all over again, I would have skipped everything but the wedding. I could have asked my husband to explain the situation to anyone who asked.

After that experience, I skipped some social occasions for the summer that I normally would have attended. **You need to do what is best for your health and physical comfort**. Give yourself a break and don't worry about what others might think. You can always explain later when talking doesn't hurt.

 "*Flying by the seat of your pants*" can be exciting and fun, but there is not going to be much excitement or fun if you are too hungry and feel too miserable to enjoy the flight.

CHAPTER 15

Routine Versus Rut

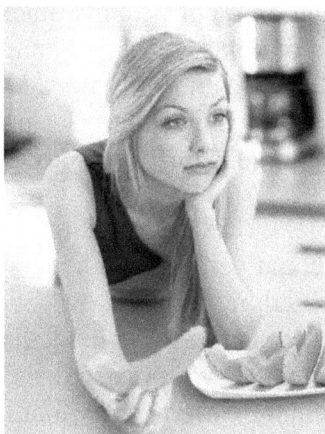

© Can Stock Photo Inc. / CITAlliance

I don't know if it was a good or a bad thing, but I had pretty much gotten into a routine a couple of weeks into my new diet.

For lunch, I would throw a couple of the bottled ready-to-go drinks in my lunch bag. It takes about nine and a half seconds to do that, so that was certainly a quick fix for the time being. One of the shakes was for mid-morning snack and the other was for my lunch.

At first that's all I was eating during the day. Those ready-made products tended to be less messy than the soups and they certainly were quicker! I didn't want to make a spectacle of myself in the lunchroom either.

There was a big problem with my quick fix, though. By the time I got home, I was SO hungry and weak-feeling that there was no time for a "Hello honey!" and a kiss. It was more like "Get out of my way because I need to get some food now!"

After a couple weeks of drinking just those two small drink containers that I had been taking to work, I started taking a huge bowl of soup to work with me, as well as the two liquid shakes. When I started doing that, it was easier to get through the day and I had more variety in my food.

It's good to have some kind of a routine to save yourself time, but you also don't want to drive yourself totally nuts by eating the same foods over and over again. Do whatever you can to "spice it up" or vary what you are eating. Even if you change a recipe by just one or two ingredients, it all helps.

CHAPTER 16

The "Unwiring/Unscrewing"

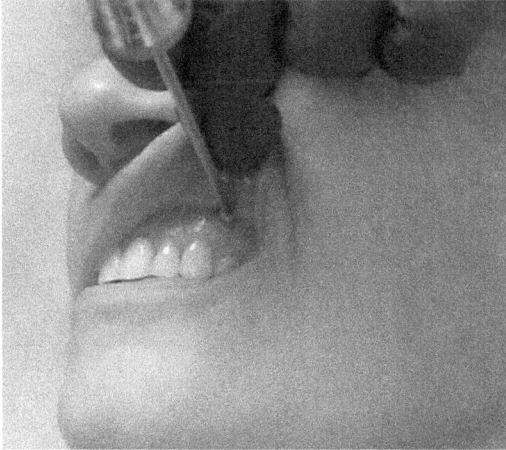

The day had finally arrived when I could have the wires and screws taken out of my mouth!

Returning my mouth to normal was actually a pretty simple process. There was no sedation involved and the whole thing only took about 45 minutes, if I remember correctly.

A simple Phillips screwdriver was used to get the screws out and a needle-nosed pliers did the unwiring.

Since it had been six weeks, my gums had started to grow around the screws in my mouth, so that part was rather uncomfortable. The good part was that with every turn of the screwdriver there was a huge release of pressure. As each screw came out, I was amazed at how good it immediately felt! When all of the screws were out, I couldn't believe how "normal" my mouth felt. There was a little bleeding, but not very much and after a very short while, there was no bleeding at all.

Below is a picture of the four screws that were in my mouth. I am so glad that I never saw them before they went into my mouth!

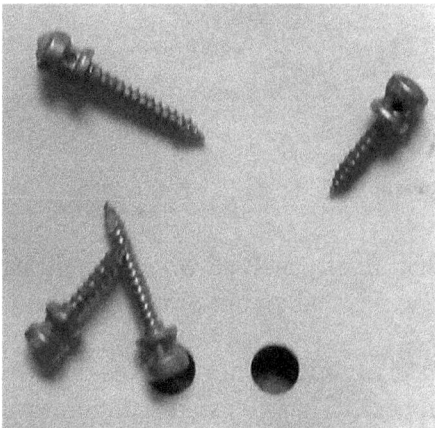

Before I left the Doctor's office that morning, I made sure to clarify what I could and could not eat.

I specifically asked about eating a cheeseburger and french fries. Luckily, they said that it was fine if my mouth wasn't too sore. (I had cased out a McDonald's that was approximately two minutes away from the Doctor's office that morning, so that's all I had been thinking about since I saw that big yellow arch!)

Remember to check with your Doctor about how your eating restrictions may or may not have changed after the fixtures are removed from your mouth.

Also, remind the Doctor what you do for work. Find out if you still have any restrictions and for how long. As I mentioned, I had been working with small children before I had my surgery. After surgery, I could not work with them while my jaws were wired. After all of the gadgets were out, I was told to wait at least another six weeks before I went back to my regular job duties.

Some jobs are not very flexible, so there is always the chance that you may not be working for some time. Maybe you will need to find another job that can accommodate your situation. **Do what you can so that everything has time to heal. Err on the side of caution!**

Back to my eating at McDonald's story...

When we got to McDonald's, it wasn't quite as I had imagined it. I had seriously thought that I would literally be inhaling my greasy fare. I didn't realize that my jaws would have so little mobility at first. So instead of "chomping" down on my food, I had to squish my burger together and take dainty small bites.

After we left McDonald's, my husband and I met two of my sisters and their spouses and we went to the Minneapolis State Fair. The process of eating

71

was slow and uncomfortable. However, that did not stop me from making some very good attempts at eating several different foods that I would not have normally eaten before this surgery. **I was very careful, though, to not bite into anything that might compromise the healing of my jawbone.**

If your jaw surgery is more extensive than mine was, you may not be able to jump back into things as quickly as I did. I considered myself quite fortunate!

CHAPTER 17

Getting Back To Normal

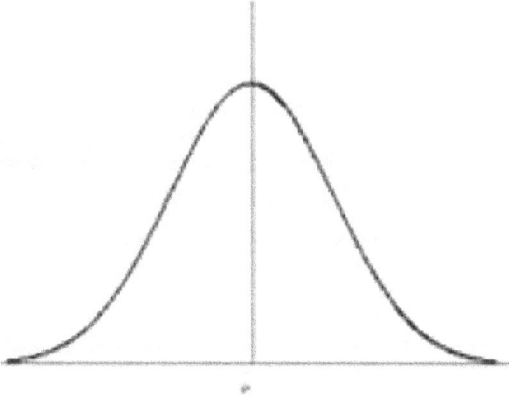

You are now at a point where everything artificial is out of your mouth. Yippee - good for you!

As I mentioned, the mobility in your jaws will definitely not be at 100% yet and eating the way you used to will not happen overnight. Your jaws and face will probably be sore too.

To help get myself back to normal, one of the things that I started working on right away was increasing my jaw mobility. I did that just by talking and doing some jaw exercises. Another thing that I frequently did was to massage the area where the screws had left small, outward dents in my face. (Of course I got the Doctor's approval for doing these things first).

Visually, there was nothing wrong with my jawbone area. However, I had been told that it would take a good year for everything to fully heal, so I knew that I still had to be careful.

Be careful of what *you* eat and what you do. The key is to work your way up – but do it gradually.

Whether it is during follow-up visits or on the phone, **don't ever hesitate to ask whether or not certain foods or certain activities are okay if you are unsure about them.**

Since we are all unique individuals, I know that this book has not covered all of the possible scenarios of your jaw surgery or the experience of being on a special diet. We are all going to have different situations and experience things differently than someone else.

However, I truly hope that this book will be "hands-on" helpful to you because I actually experienced the things that I wrote about.

I was "there" and I hope that I helped you.

Thanks for Reading!

Your feedback would be much appreciated. If you found this book to be helpful or would like to offer some constructive criticism, feel free to send an email to: djflaagan@gra.midco.net.

I would also really appreciate it if you would be kind enough to leave a review at Amazon for me at:

Amazon Book Review

Sincerely,

Jayne Flaagan